HEALTHKINS EXERCISE!

by Jane Belk Moncure
illustrated by Helen Endres

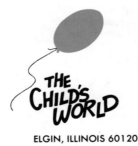

THE CHILD'S WORLD

ELGIN, ILLINOIS 60120

Distributed by Childrens Press, 1224 West Van Buren Street,
Chicago, Illinois 60607.

Library of Congress Cataloging in Publication Data

Moncure, Jane Belk.
    Healthkins exercise!

    Summary: The Healthkins demonstrate all the different
kinds of exercise that will make them, and us, feel
good and stay healthy.
    1. Exercise—Juvenile literature.   [1. Exercise.
2. Health]   I. Endres, Helen, ill.   II. Title.
RA781.M615   1982   613.7'1   82-14712
ISBN 0-89565-241-2

1 2 3 4 5 6 7 8 9 10 11 12 R 89 88 87 86 85 84 83 82

HEALTHKINS EXERCISE!

Come on in.
Join the fun.
Exercises have begun.

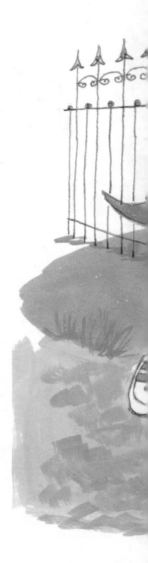

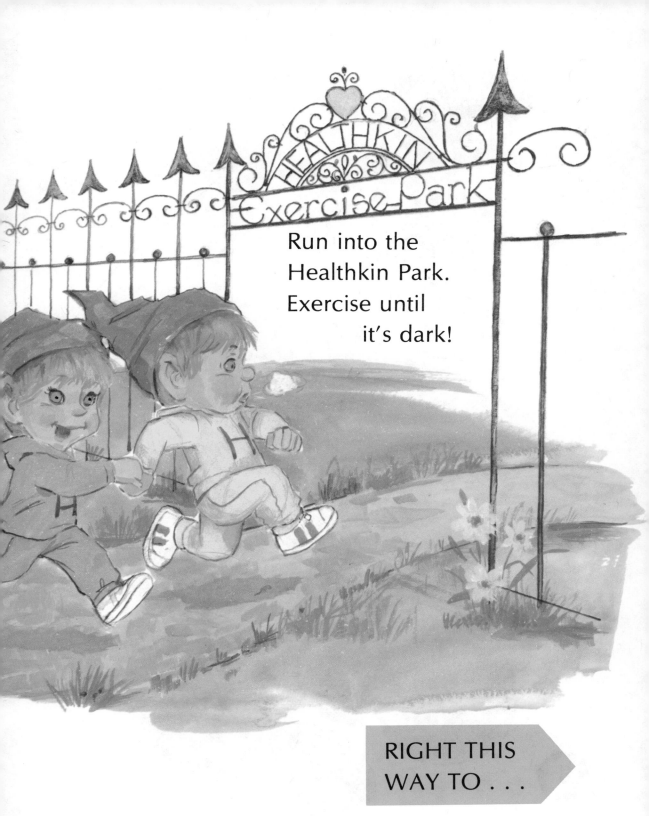

Run into the
Healthkin Park.
Exercise until
it's dark!

RIGHT THIS
WAY TO . . .

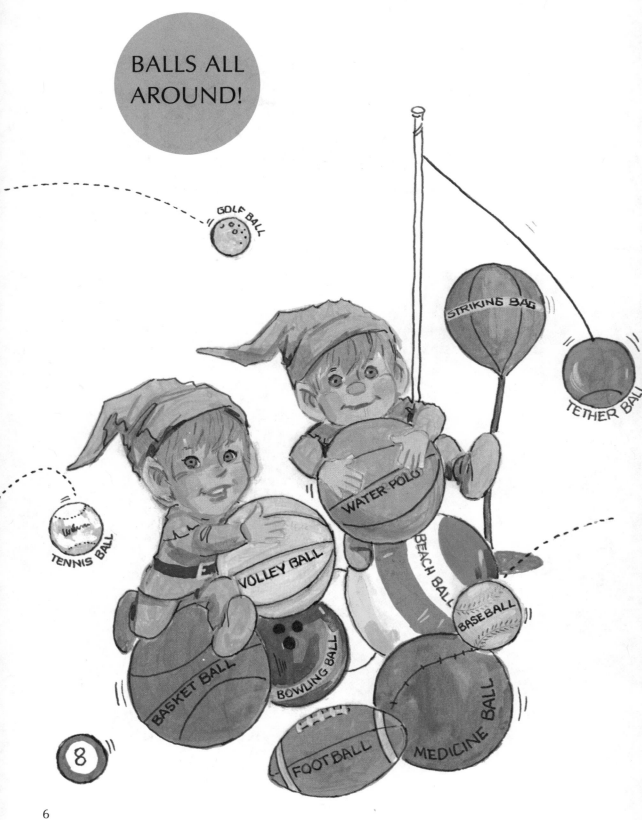

BALLS ALL AROUND!

Healthkins pitch . . .

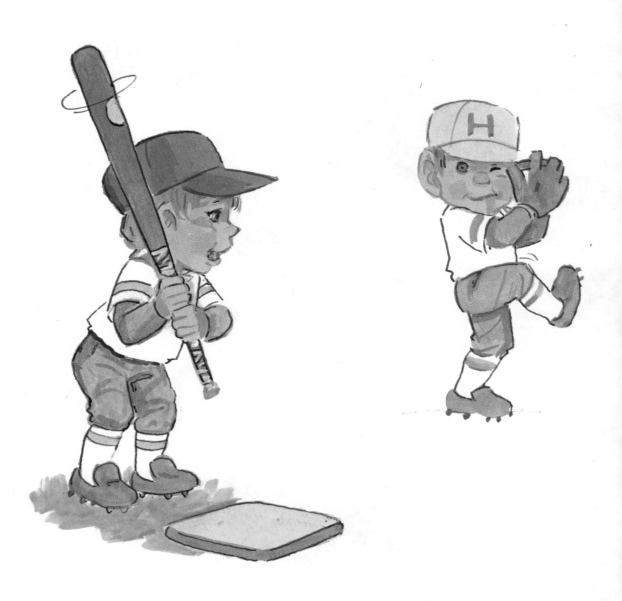

and bat . . .

. . . catch . . .

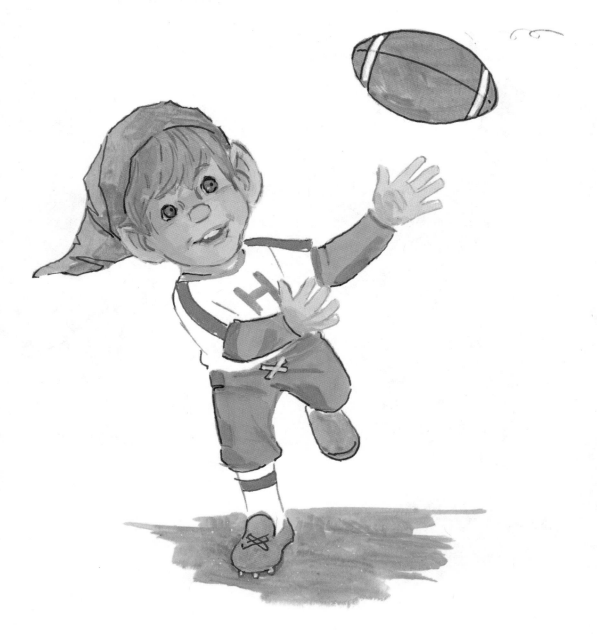

and throw.
Playing ball helps Healthkins grow!

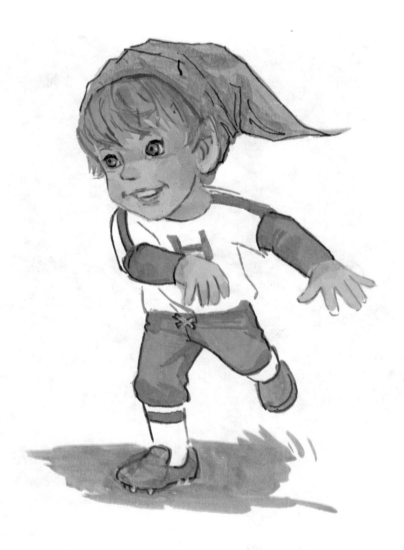

It can help you, too.

HEAD
FOR . . .

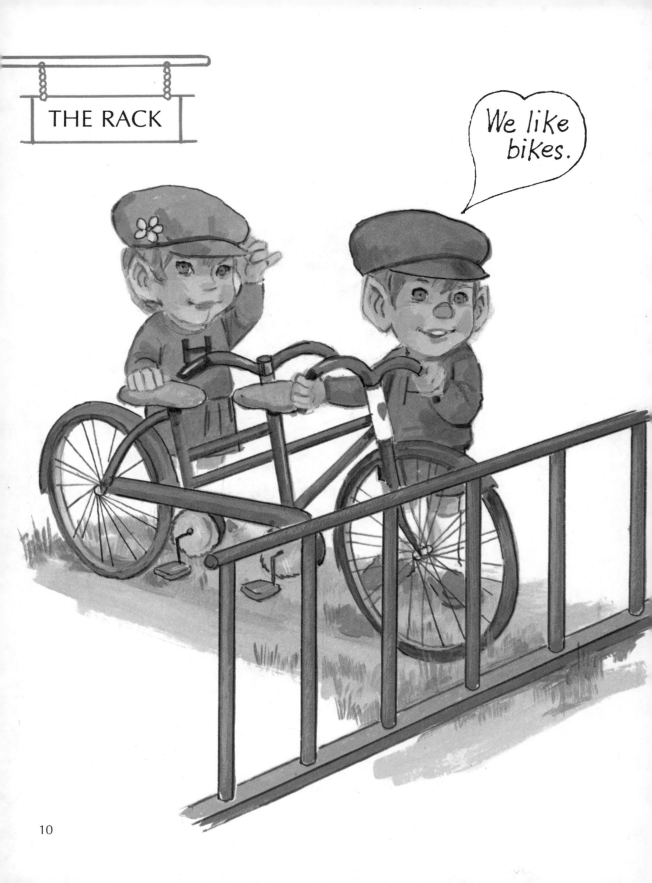

Some Healthkins ride bikes all day long.
They know bike riding makes them strong!

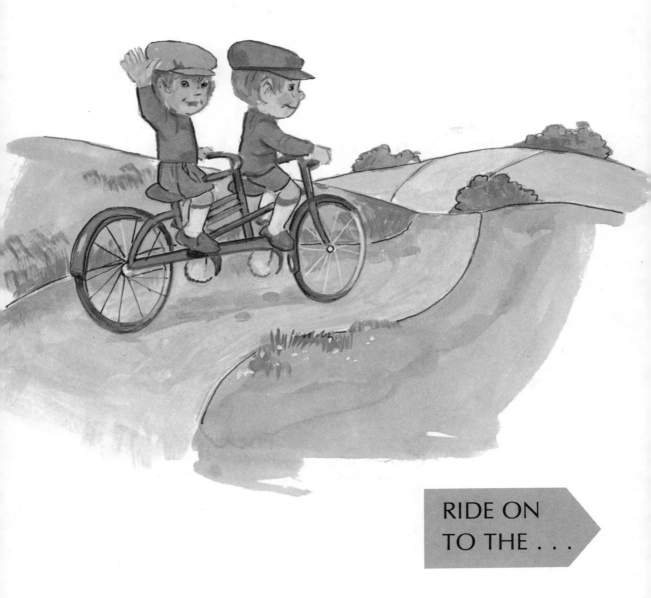

RIDE ON
TO THE . . .

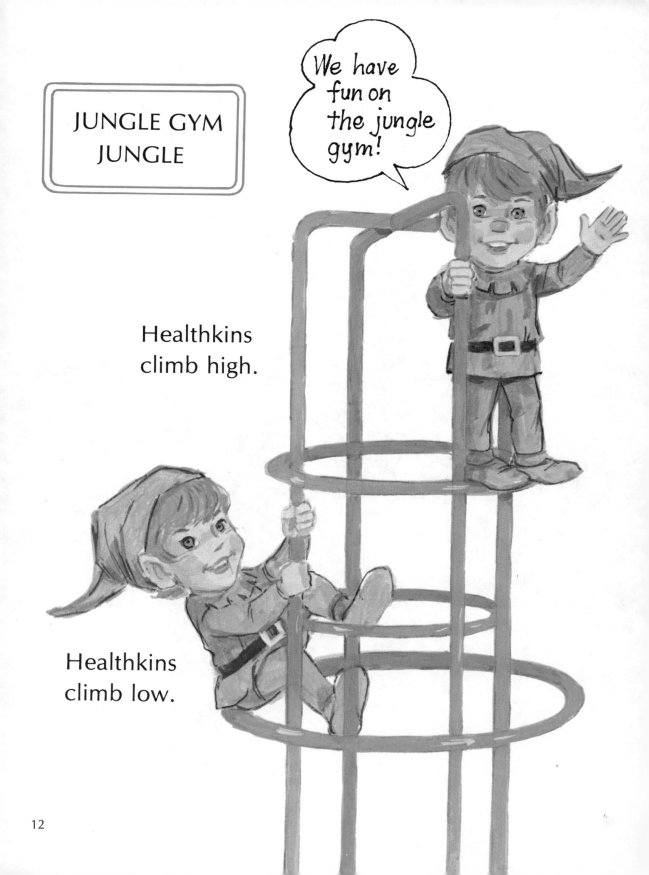

Climbing helps them stretch and grow.

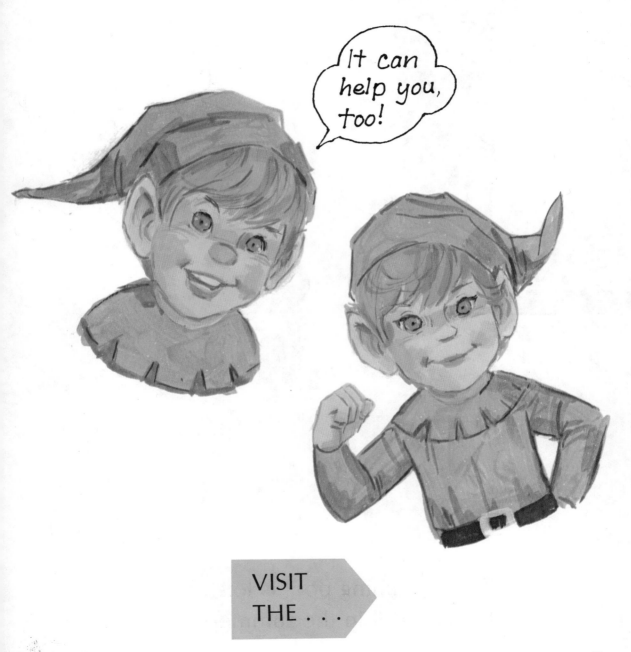

VISIT
THE . . .

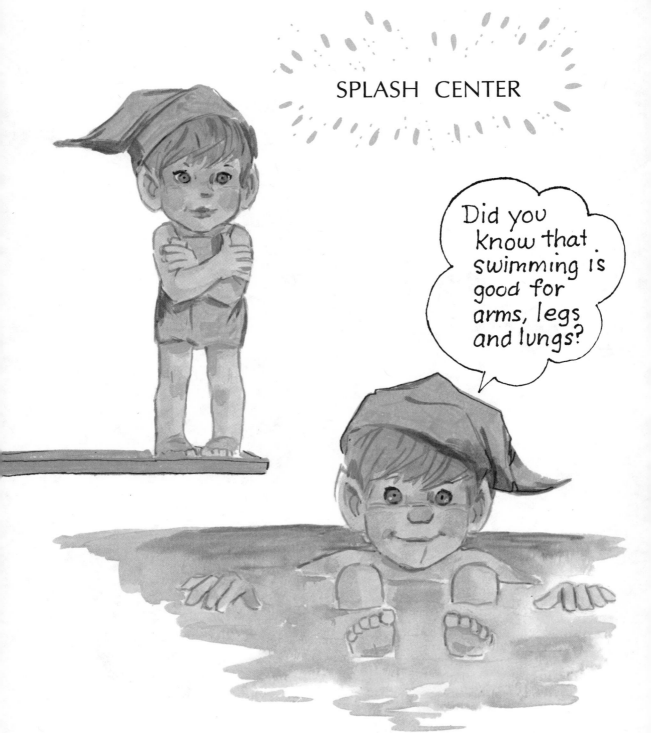

SPLASH CENTER

Did you know that swimming is good for arms, legs and lungs?

The swimming pool is lots of fun.
It feels cool in the summer sun!

Follow the Healthkins!
Do as they do.

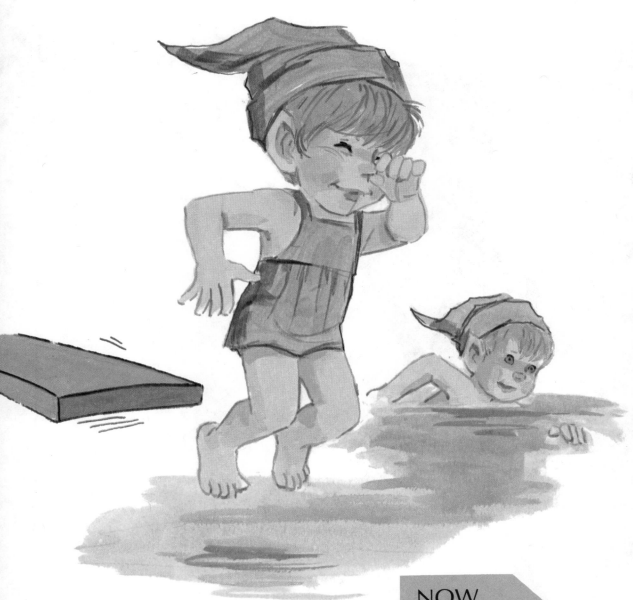

Swimming helps them.
And it can help you!

NOW
JOIN . . .

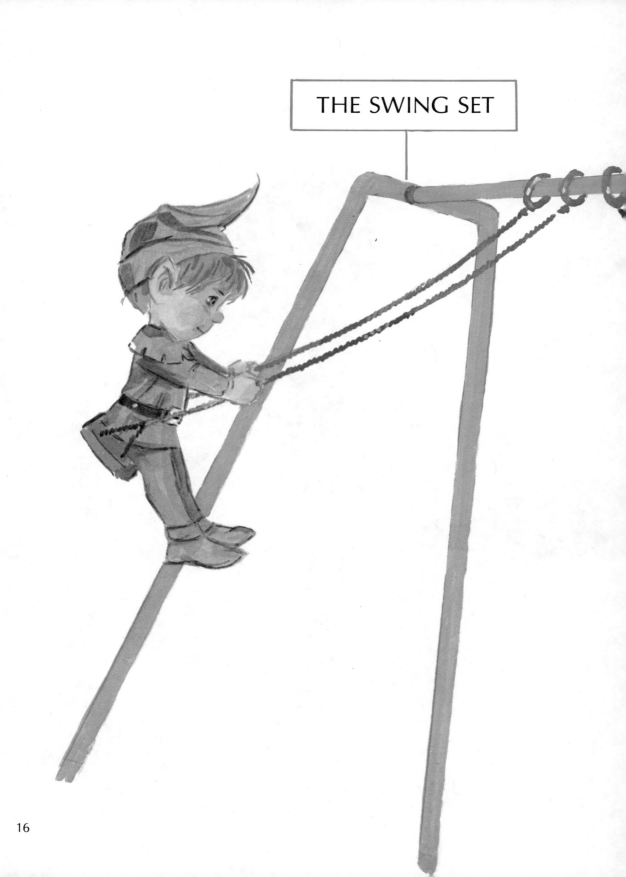

THE SWING SET

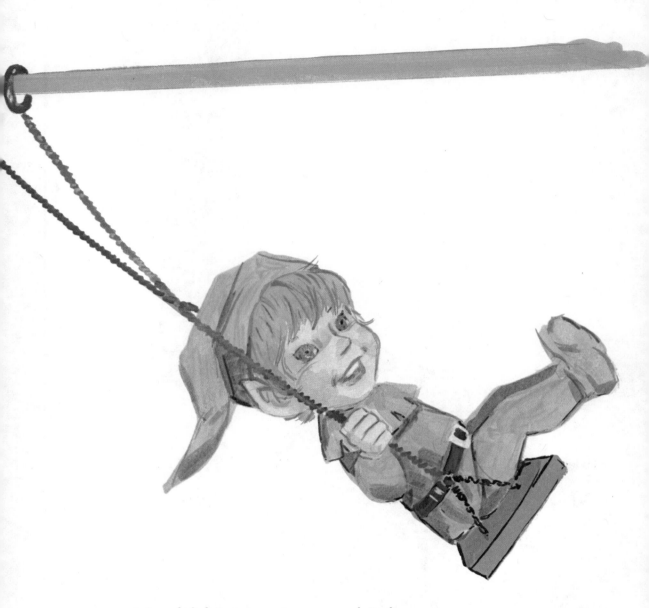

Healthkins swing up high.
They swing down low.
Pumping helps their muscles grow.

This park has walks
to skate on,

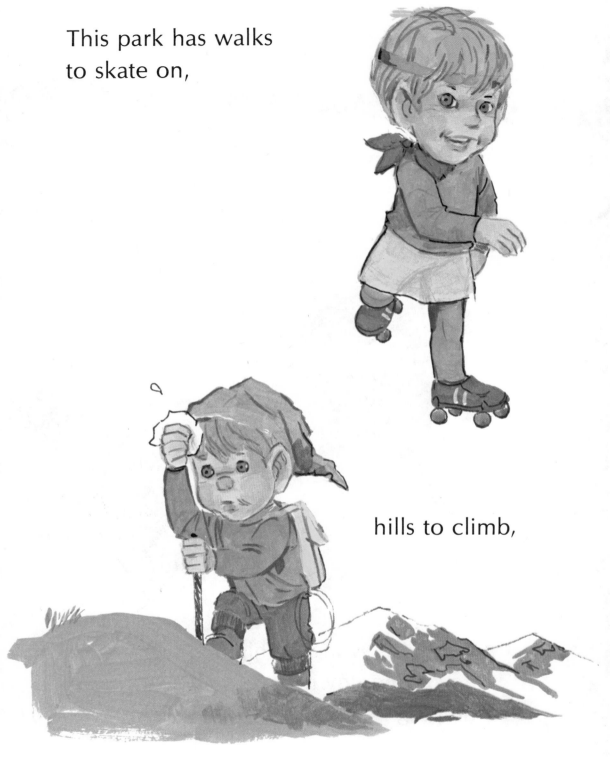

hills to climb,

18

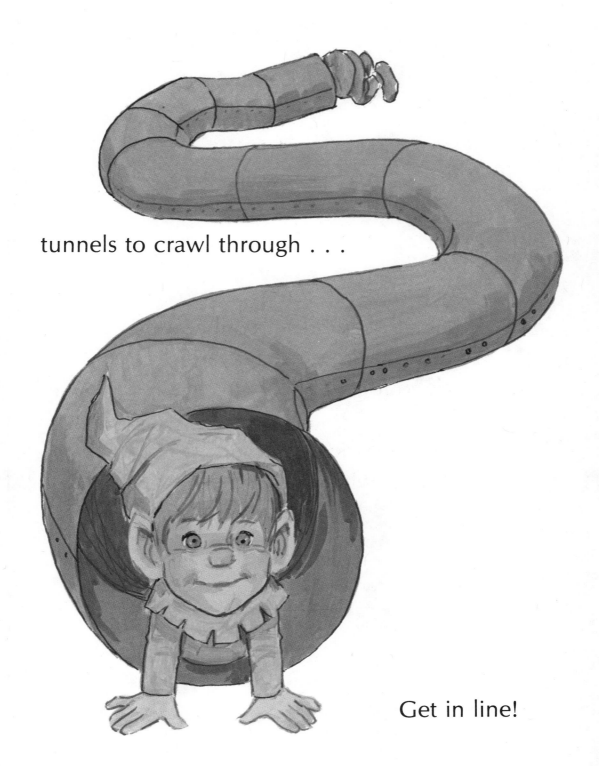

tunnels to crawl through . . .

Get in line!

Healthkin Parks are all around.
Just check your backyard
or your school playground.

Pick a park that's right for you.
That is what the Healthkins do!

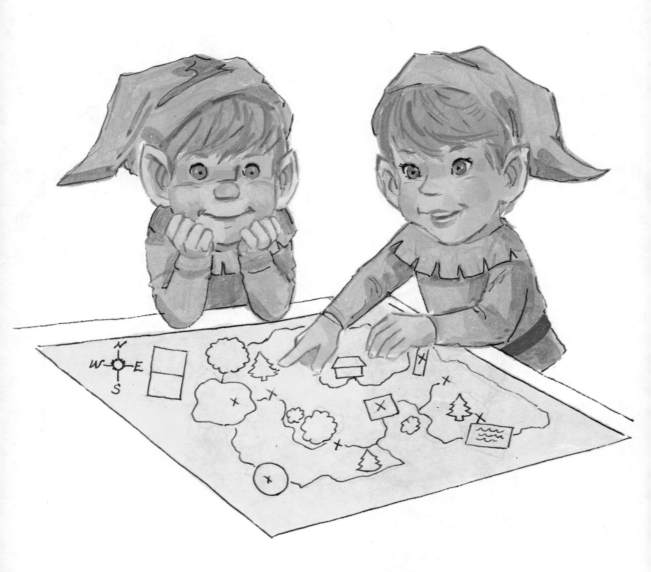

Healthkins have strong muscles because . . .

they hop,

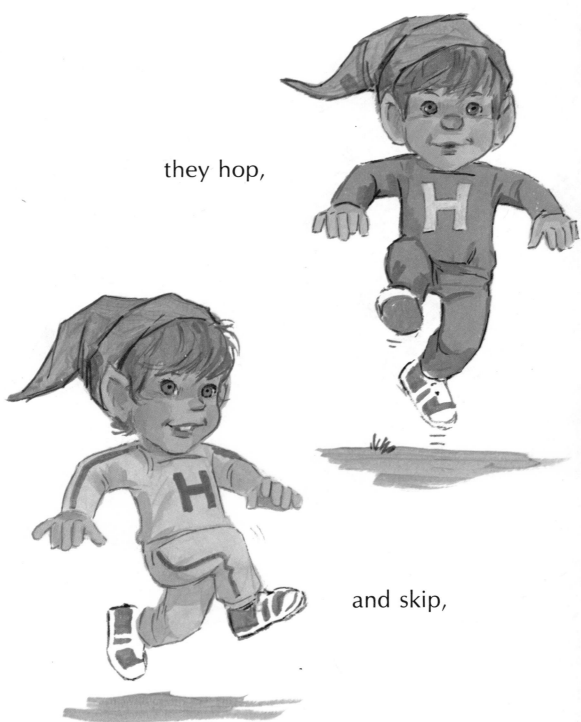

and skip,

and walk,

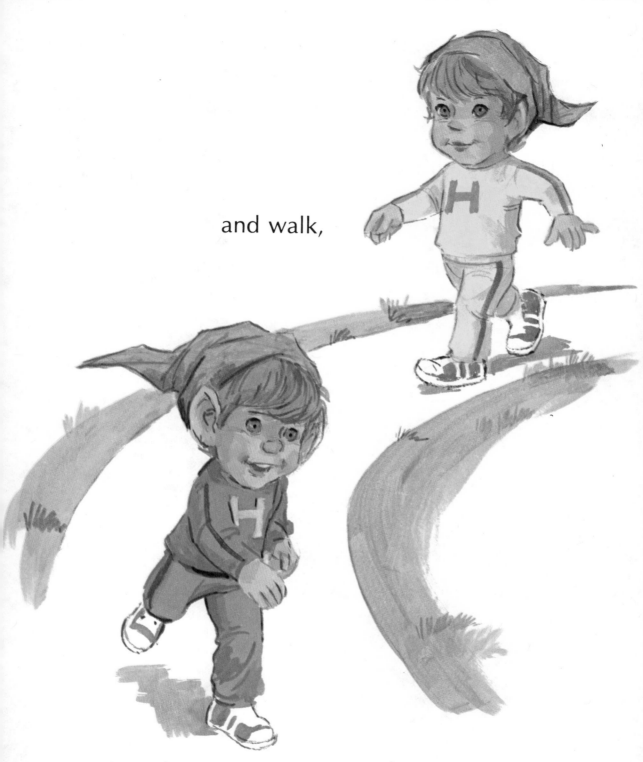

and jog.

They stretch up high . . .

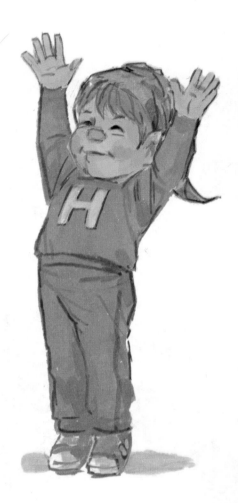

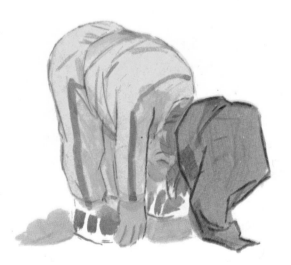

and bend down low . . .

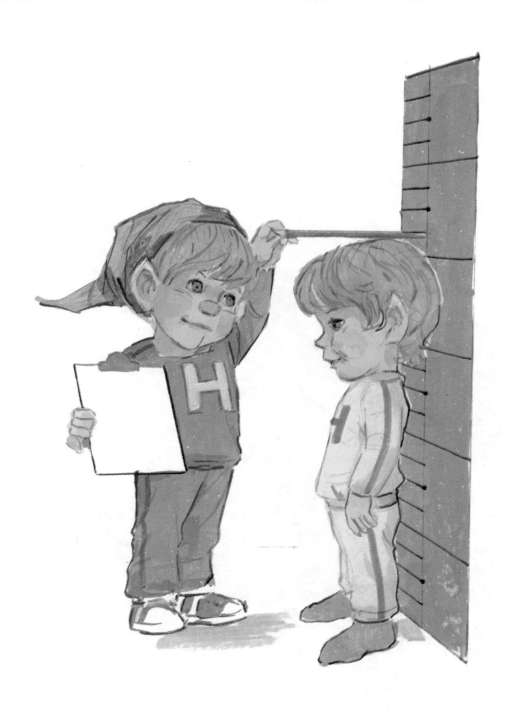

exercising as they grow.

Once a week, Healthkins sit—

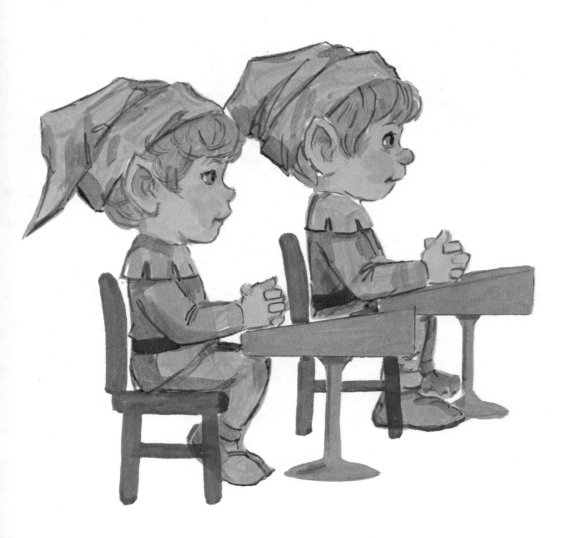

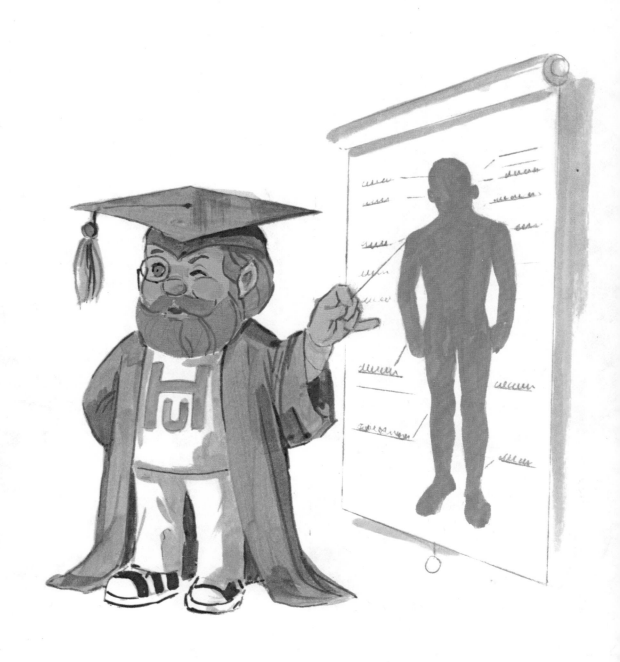

to take a class called, ''Keeping Fit.''

Then, after class,
when work is done,

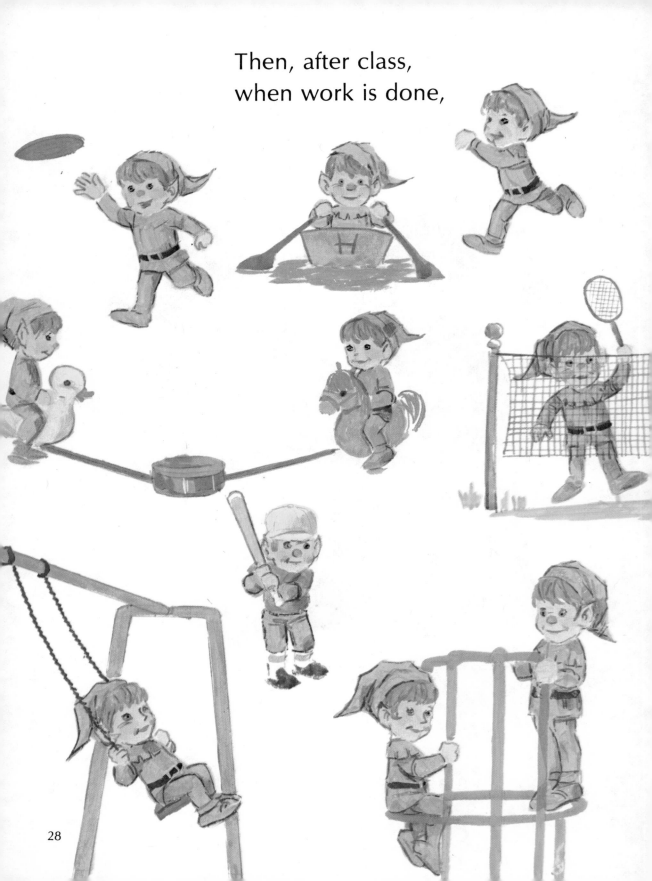

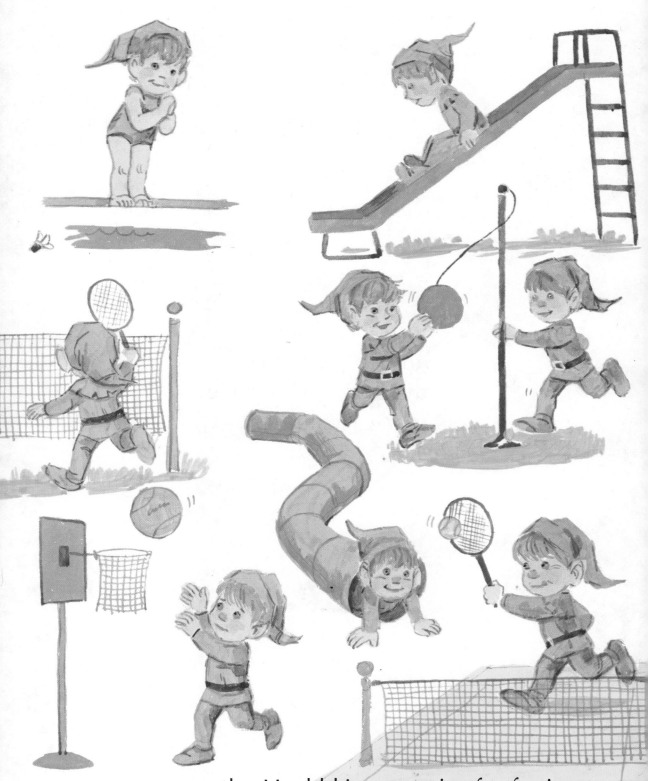

the Healthkins exercise for fun!

Just do as they do,
and you may win—
the Happy Healthkin,
Good Health Pin!

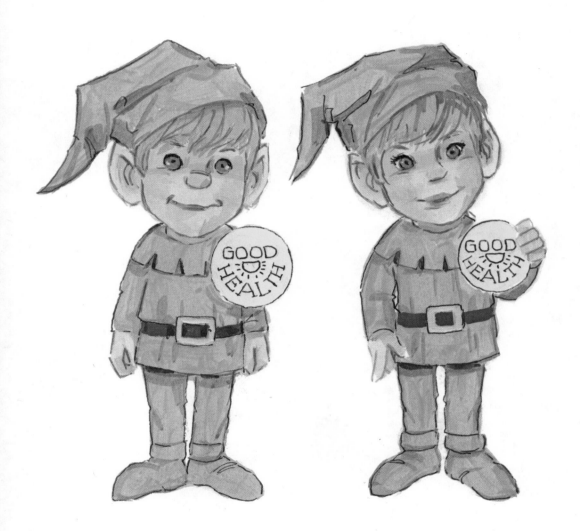